MENTAL HEALTH GUIDES

UNDERSTANDING ADDICTION

by Heather C. Hudak

BrightPoint Press

San Diego, CA

BrightPoint Press

an imprint of ReferencePoint Press, Inc.
Printed in the United States

For more information, contact:
BrightPoint Press
PO Box 27779
San Diego, CA 92198
www.BrightPointPress.com

Content Consultant: Michael J. Zvolensky, PhD; Hugh Roy and Lillie Cranz Cullen Distinguished University Professor; Director, Anxiety and Health Research Laboratory/Substance Use Treatment Clinic, University of Houston

LIBRARY OF CONGRESS CATALOGING-IN-PUBLICATION DATA

Names: Hudak, Heather C., 1975- author.
Title: Understanding addiction / Heather C. Hudak.
Description: San Diego : ReferencePoint Press, 2021. | Series: Mental health guides | Includes bibliographical references and index. | Audience: Grades 10-12
Identifiers: LCCN 2020002444 (print) | LCCN 2020002445 (eBook) | ISBN 9781682829813 (hardcover) | ISBN 9781682829820 (eBook)
Subjects: LCSH: Compulsive behavior--Juvenile literature. | Compulsive behavior--Treatment--Juvenile literature.
Classification: LCC RC533 .H83 2020 (print) | LCC RC533 (eBook) | DDC 616.85/84--dc23
LC record available at https://lccn.loc.gov/2020002444
LC eBook record available at https://lccn.loc.gov/2020002445

CONTENTS

AT A GLANCE

- Addiction is a long-term issue. It can take many years for people to overcome an addiction. Some people are addicted to substances. They may have a substance use disorder (SUD). Others are addicted to certain behaviors.
- There are several types of SUDs. Nicotine addiction is the most common.
- There are many signs and symptoms of addiction. The most common symptom is cravings. The person has a constant and powerful need for the substance.
- More than two percent of people around the world have an SUD. Many things contribute to addiction. Some people's brains respond more to a substance. Family history and environment can play a role too.

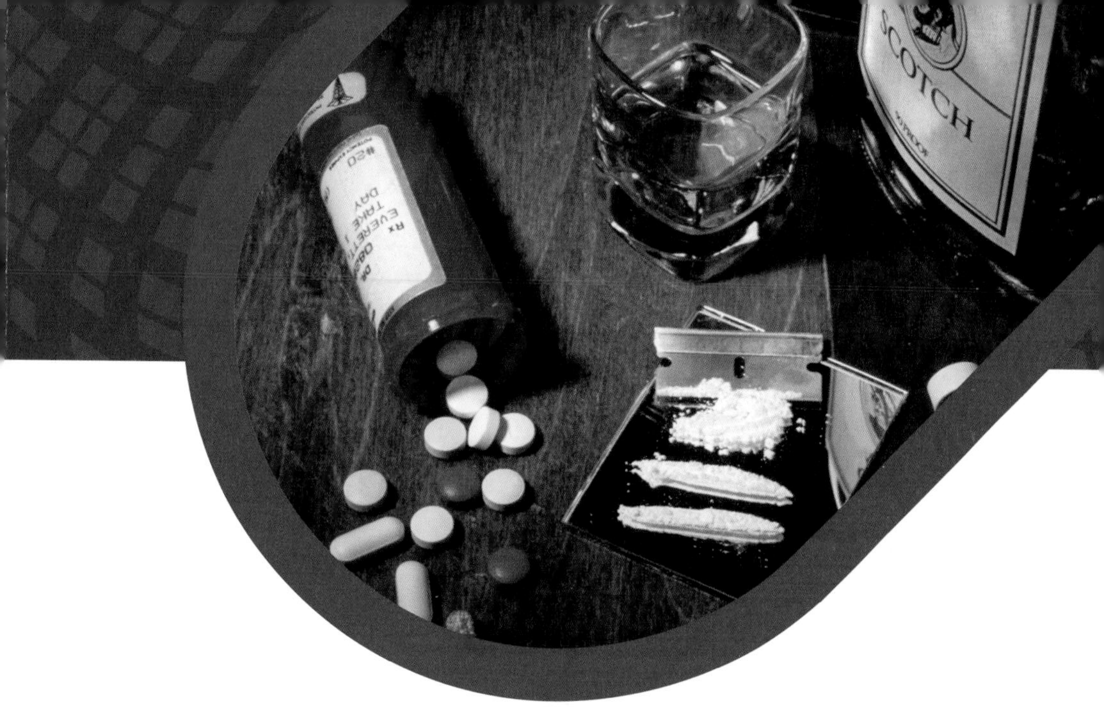

- Substance abuse can cause health problems. Health issues from substance abuse caused nearly 12 million deaths in 2017.

- More than 20 million Americans over the age of twelve have an SUD. But only about 10 percent get the help they need.

- There is no cure for addiction. But it can be treated.

THE PATH TO ADDICTION

Alex was a Boy Scout. He played sports. He had a good relationship with his family. Then he made a decision that changed his life. Alex was thirteen years old when he first tried **cannabis**. He was just starting middle school. Some of his friends smoked cannabis. Alex wanted to see what he was missing.

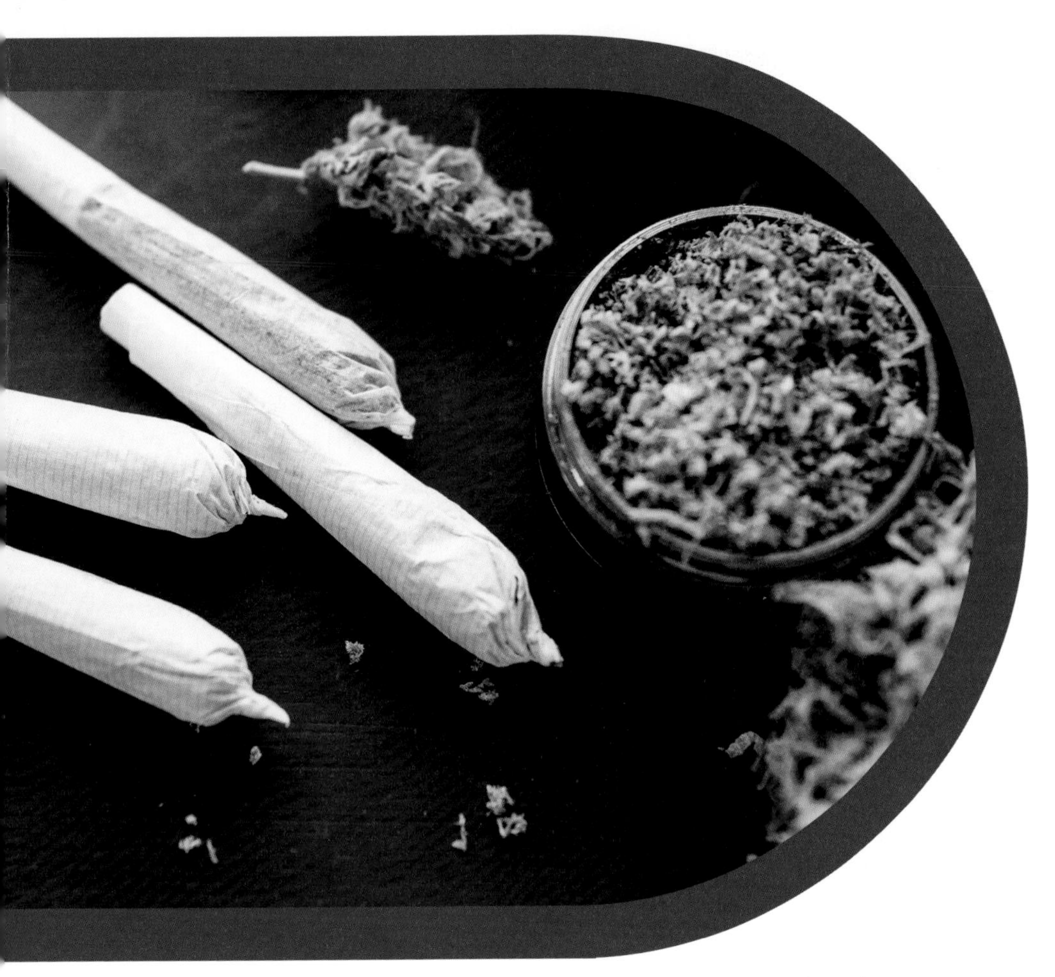

Cannabis is one of the most widely used drugs in the United States.

Soon Alex was using cannabis daily. He started using other drugs too. He used any substance he could get his hands on. He began drinking alcohol when he was fifteen.

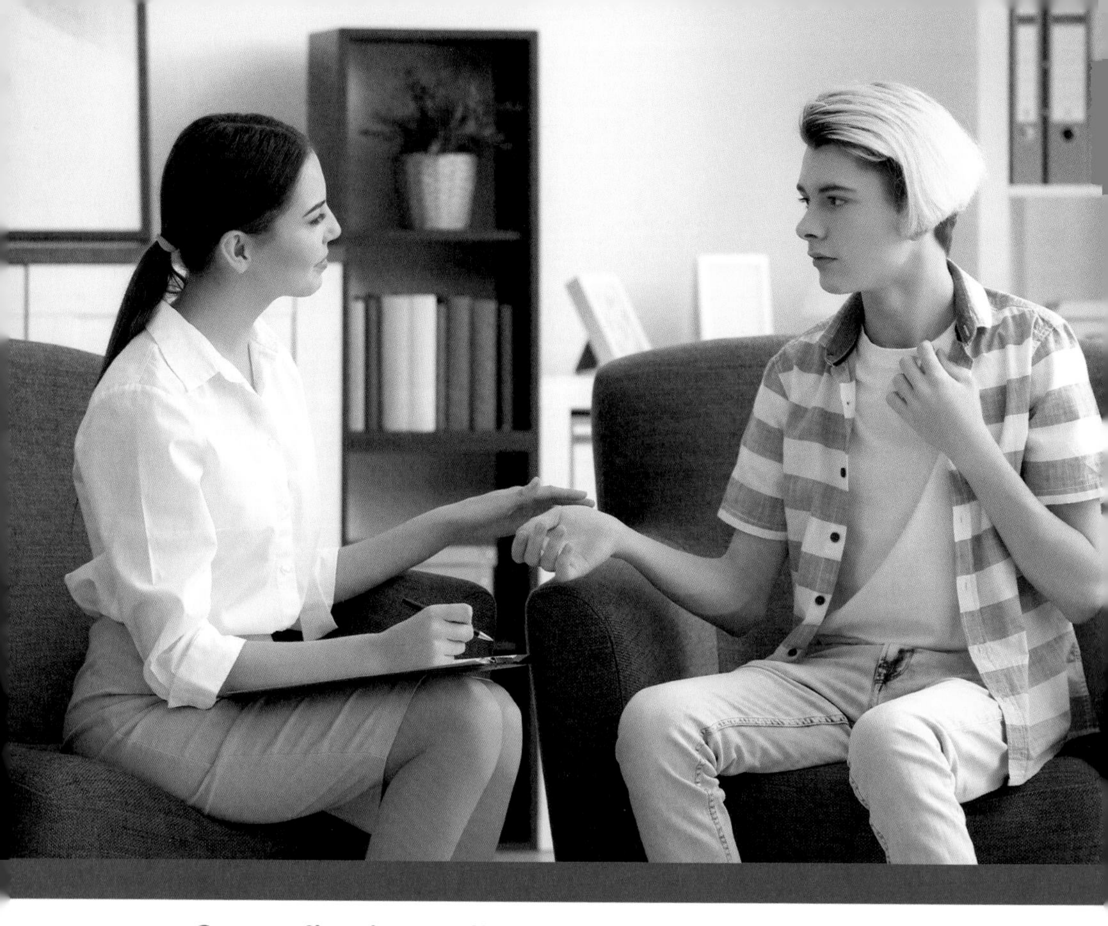

Counseling is an effective treatment for many types of addiction.

He took his father's pain pills. He started using heroin at the age of seventeen.

Alex needed drugs to get through each day. He used drugs at school. He needed money to buy more drugs. So he stole money from his family.

Finally, Alex told his parents that he was using drugs. They took him to see a counselor. Alex lied and said he was getting better. He said he was no longer using drugs. But he was still using them every day.

Alex's grades began to slip. He worried that he would not be able to graduate. His relationship with his family became strained. Alex finally decided to stop using drugs. He said, "It was like something just clicked in my brain and I knew—I can't keep doing this or I'm going to die."[1]

Alex asked for help to overcome his addiction. He started treatment on his eighteenth birthday. He stopped using substances. Then he went to live at a treatment center for a while. He began to get better. Over time, his family started to trust him again. They grew closer than ever before.

Finally, Alex was able to leave the treatment center. He went back to finish high school. He got a job. He applied to college. He wanted to become a drug and

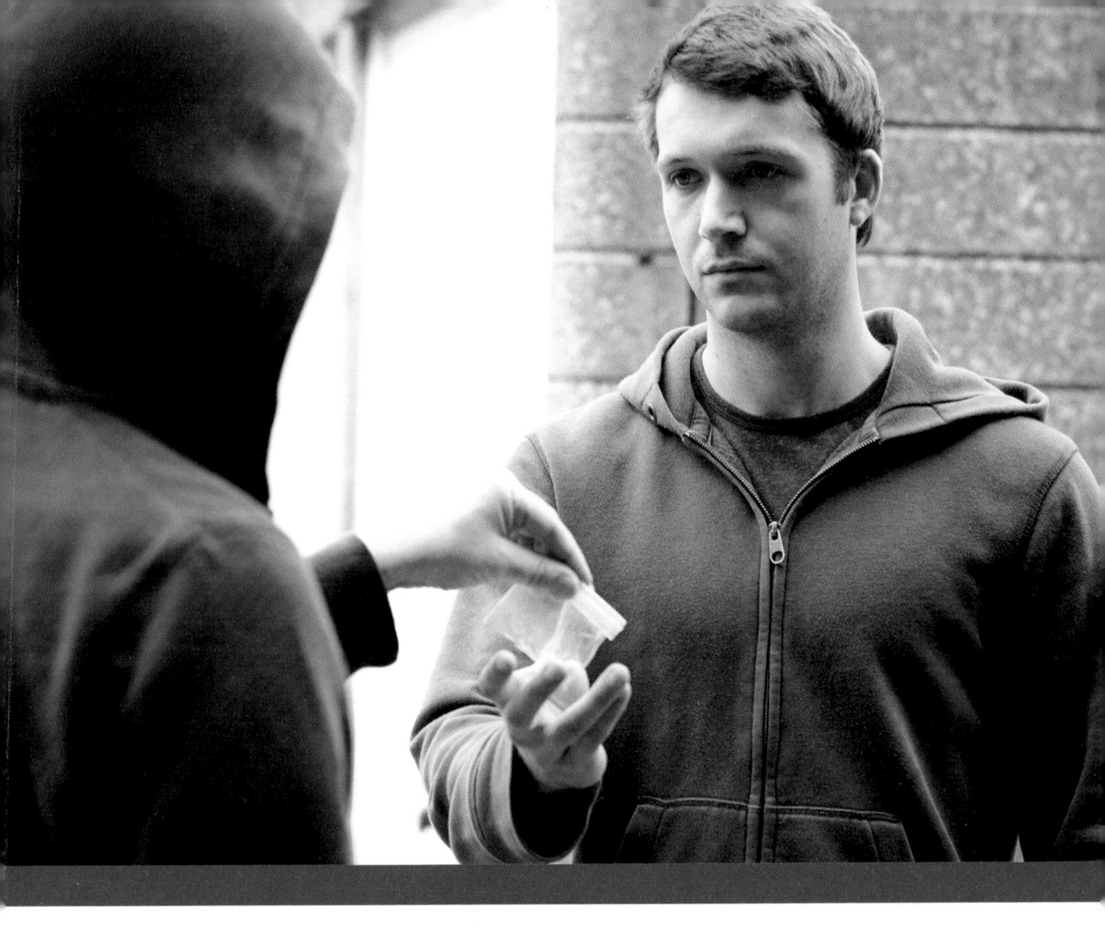

People who first use drugs as teenagers are at a high risk for becoming addicted.

alcohol counselor. As a counselor, he could help others who had addictions. Alex had learned how to cope with his addiction. He found ways to be happy without using drugs.

CHAPTER ONE

WHAT IS ADDICTION?

Addiction is difficult to overcome. People may have an addiction for many years. Many people have substance use disorders (SUDs). They are addicted to drugs or alcohol. This is the most common type of addiction. People get pleasure from using these substances. This feeling is

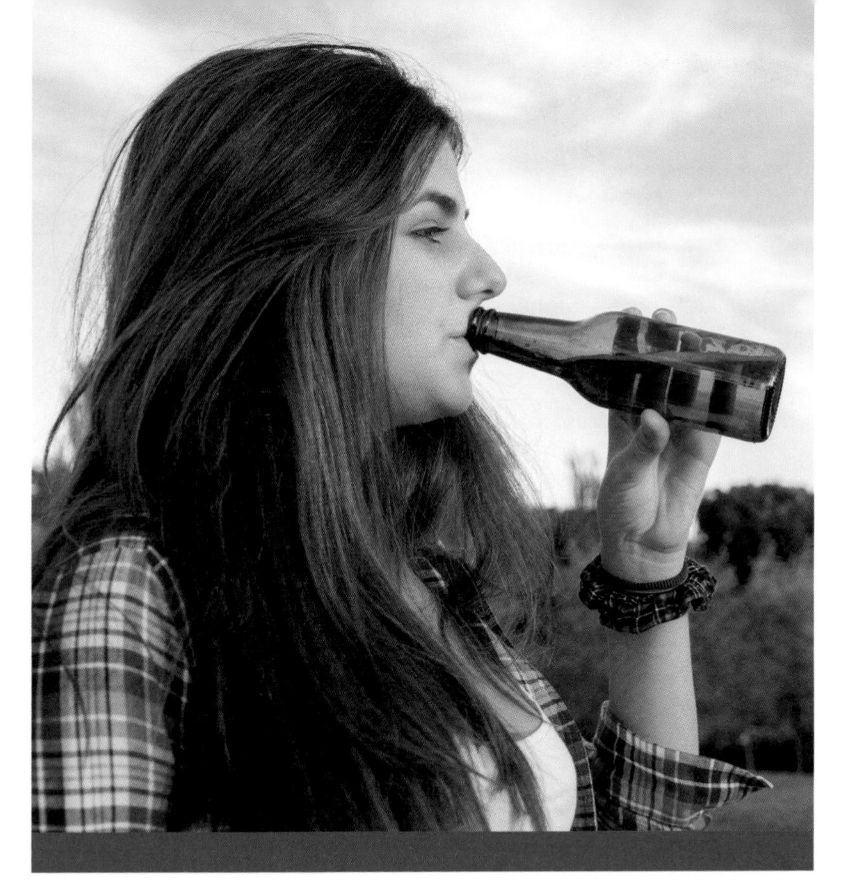

Most medical groups consider addiction to be a disease because of the changes it causes in a person's brain.

called a high. People will do anything to get this high.

It is very hard to stop an addiction. Sal Raichbach is a psychologist. He treats people who have addictions. He says, "An [addicted person] doesn't just crave the drug; their body is functioning as if it cannot live without it."[2]

Addiction can become more severe over time. People can build a **tolerance**. This means they need more of a substance to get the same effects.

WHAT ARE COMPULSIONS?

Compulsions are a large part of addictions. A compulsion is a strong urge to do something. Giving into this urge causes someone a feeling of relief. But this feeling lasts only a short time. Then the person has the urge to do the behavior again. The person knows the behavior is unhealthy. But he or she does it anyway.

Substance abuse can harm a person's health. For example, drinking a lot of alcohol can cause liver damage. Drugs alter people's moods and emotions. People cannot think clearly. They may not consider the effects of their actions.

TYPES OF ADDICTION

There are several types of SUDs. Nicotine addiction is the most common. Nicotine is a substance in tobacco products. Cigarettes contain this substance. The more nicotine people use, the more they want it.

People can also develop a nicotine addiction from vaping. Vaping involves

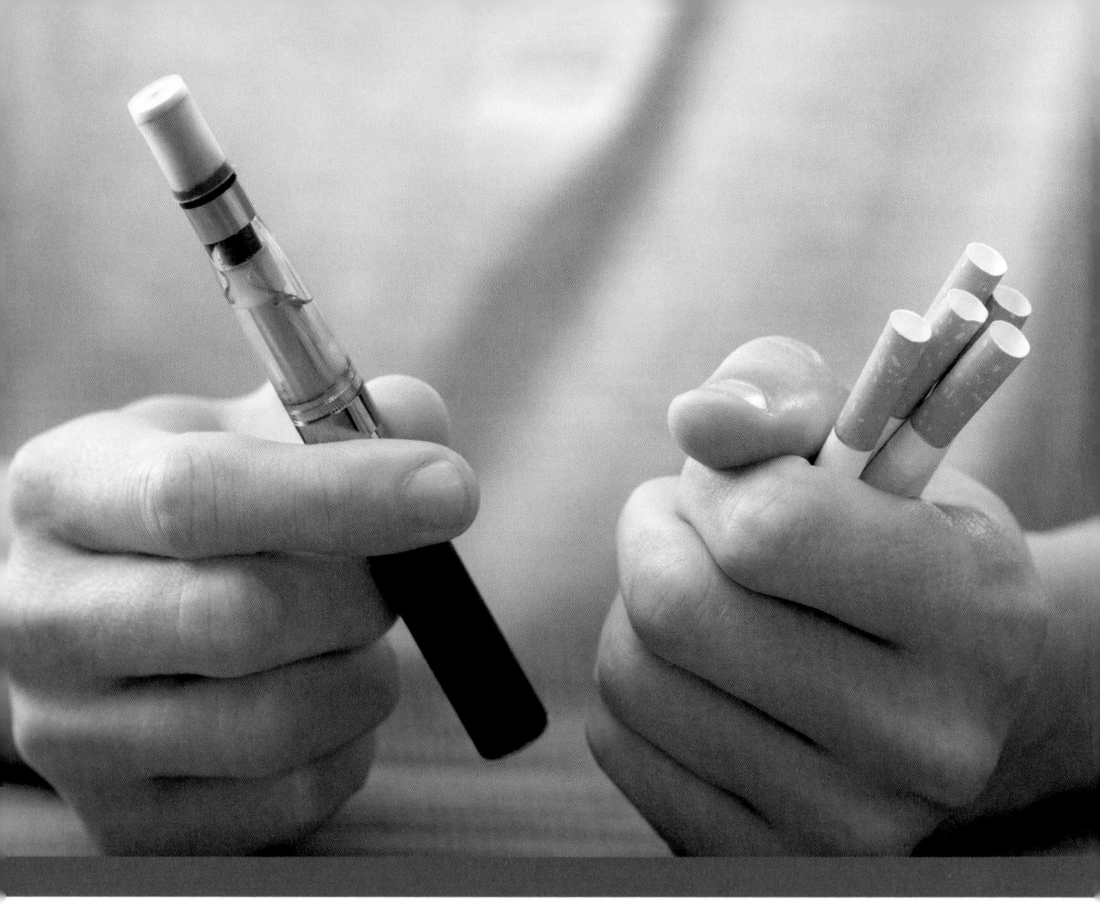

E-cigarette use is growing among teens and young adults. In 2019, 28 percent of high schoolers reported vaping nicotine in the past month.

inhaling vapor through a device, such as an e-cigarette. Many people think vaping is less addictive than smoking. But this is not always true. Most vaping products contain nicotine. Robin Koval leads the nonprofit group Truth Initiative. This group's goal is to stop the use of tobacco products. Koval says, "Some [vaping products] contain a lot [of nicotine]. . . . As these products have developed, they have become more effective at delivering nicotine."[3]

Alcoholism is the second most common type of addiction. It happens when people drink large amounts of alcohol often. This habit interferes with their daily lives. They may drink while at work or in school. Many try to hide their drinking from others.

Many people are addicted to illegal drugs. These include cocaine and heroin.

Methamphetamine (meth) is another dangerous drug. These substances affect how the brain works. They change the way a person thinks and acts. Some illegal drugs are made with strong ingredients. They have a more powerful effect. This effect also depends on how much and how often someone uses the drugs.

USE, MISUSE, AND ABUSE

Some people misuse prescription drugs. They may use more than was prescribed. They may take a drug that was prescribed to someone else. Misuse turns into abuse when people become addicted. They take the drug regularly. They also take it in large doses. Drug abuse can have harmful effects over time.

Opioids can be addictive too. Opioids are painkillers. Some are **prescription** drugs. Doctors may prescribe opioids to people who are in pain. These drugs help people feel better. But some people misuse them. They take more than they need. They may take the drug more often than they should. They may become addicted.

Not all addictions are an SUD. Some people have behavioral addictions. They feel an urge to do a certain action over and over again. They cannot control this urge. For example, eating food is an action. It makes people feel happy and full. But some people regularly eat too much food. They do not stop eating when they are full. They know is not good for them. They often feel guilty afterward. But they cannot stop. They have binge-eating disorder. Gambling is another common behavioral addiction.

WHAT CAUSES AN ADDICTION?

Not all people who try a substance develop an addiction. Some people just try a substance once. They may never try it again. Or if they do, they may be able to stop at any time. But some people's brains have a different response to the substance. They feel a stronger high. They crave

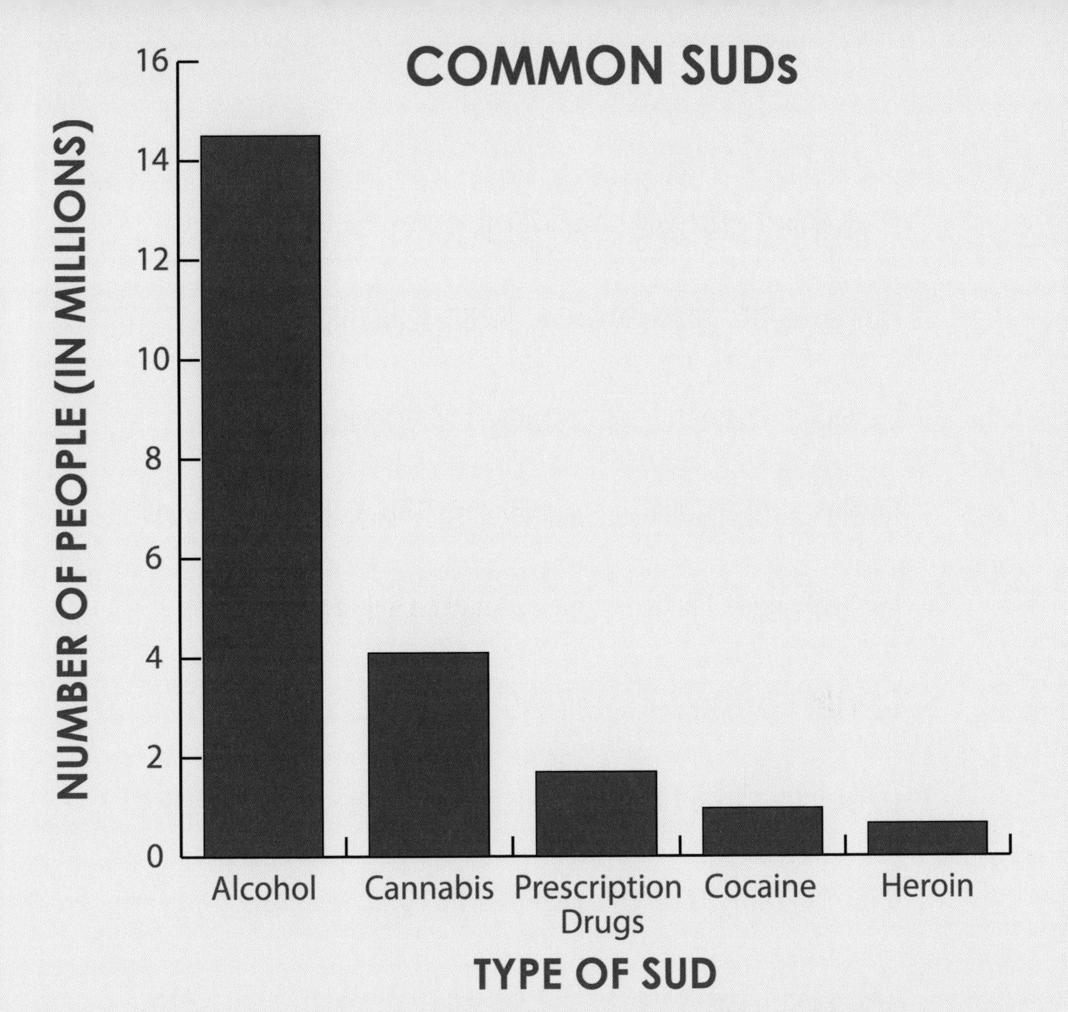

There are many types of addictions, including to both legal and illegal substances.

more of the substance. This can happen even after trying the substance only once. Nicotine or heroin are two examples of this.

Many people use drugs to help them cope with a problem. For example, some people have depression. Depression is a feeling of intense sadness. People also feel hopeless. They may abuse substances to numb these feelings. Substances may provide short-term relief. But they can make the symptoms of mental illness worse. People need to keep using the substances to feel better. They develop addictions.

Young people are more prone to addiction than older people. Some people have a family history of addiction. They are more likely to develop an addiction than those who do not have this history. A person's friend group can play a role too. For example, some people have friends who use drugs. Their friends' behaviors can influence them. They are more likely to start using drugs.

THE OPIOID CRISIS

Heroin is an illegal opioid. Other opioids are prescription drugs. They include morphine and oxycodone. Doctors may prescribe them. About 29 percent of Americans who are prescribed these drugs abuse them. People can die from this. Opioids slow a person's heart rate. The person's breathing also slows. In 2018 nearly 130 Americans died each day from opioid abuse.

CHAPTER TWO

HOW DOES ADDICTION AFFECT PEOPLE?

People go through four stages before they develop an SUD. Some people move quickly through the stages. Others move through them more slowly. An addiction may take years to develop. Spotting the signs early is important.

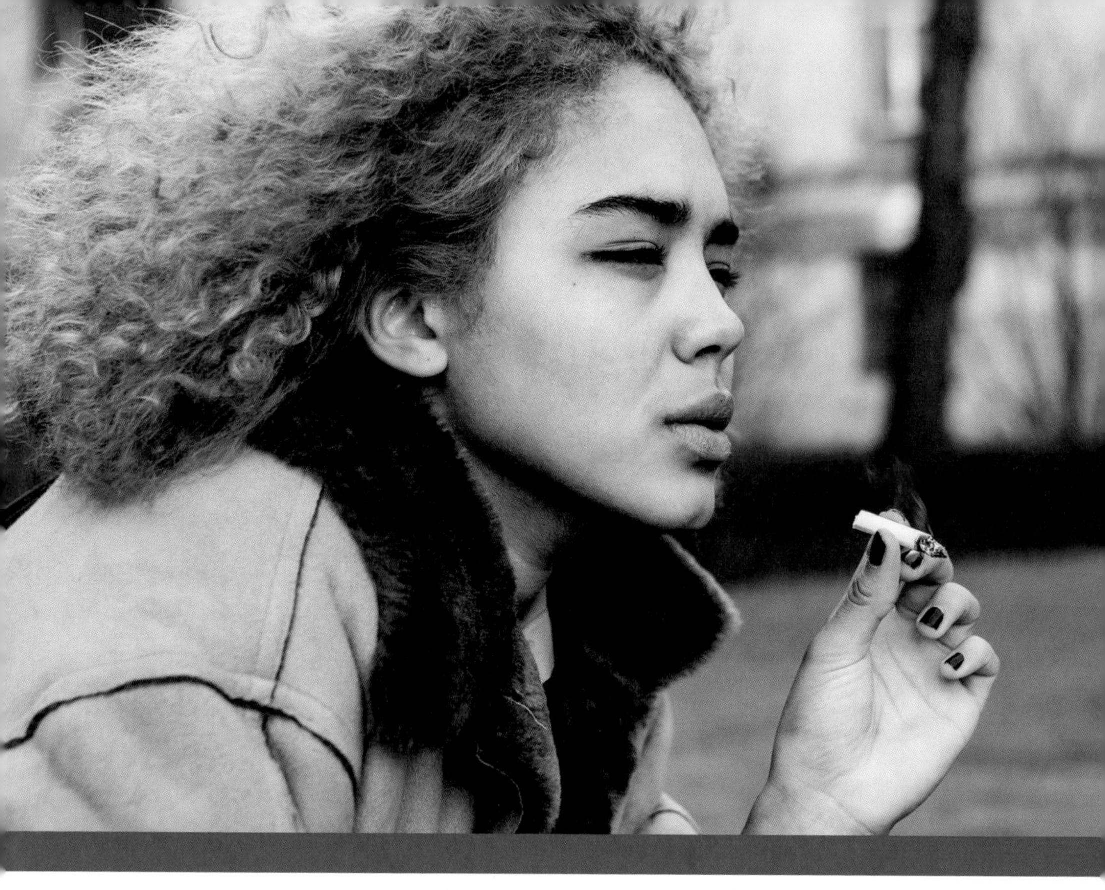

Some drugs are more powerful than others. A person may develop an addiction to these drugs very quickly.

This can help stop substance abuse before it becomes an addiction.

The first stage of substance addiction is experimentation. People experiment with

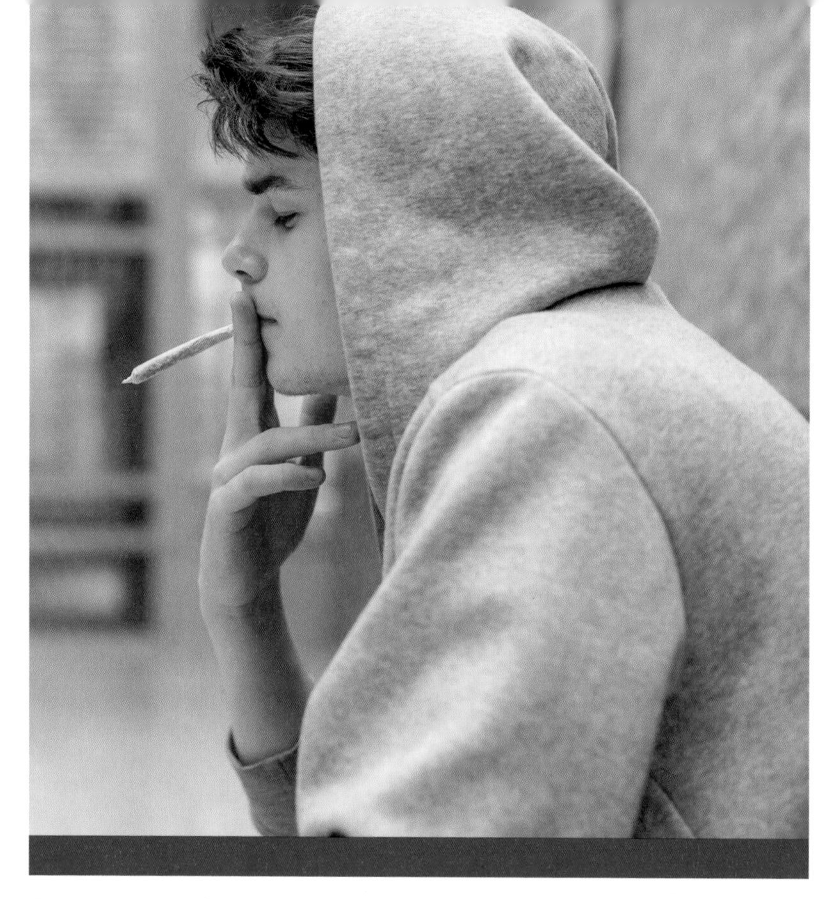

Many people who are addicted to drugs believe they can stop using substances at any time or without help.

a substance. They try the substance for the first time. Most people at this stage do not develop an addiction. They may only use the substance occasionally. They feel in control of this behavior. They can stop using the substance at any time. They may not have the desire to use it again. Others have a strong urge to continue using it. They are at risk of developing an addiction. The American Academy of Child and Adolescent Psychiatry studies mental health issues. It says, "It is difficult to know which teens will experiment and stop and which will develop serious problems."[4]

The second stage is the regular use of a substance. People at this stage start to use the substance more often. Their use becomes predictable. For example, they may start to use it every weekend. Or they may always use it when they feel a certain way, such as bored or **stressed**. This behavior becomes a habit.

The risk of addiction is much greater for people who regularly use a substance. Dennis Henigan works at the Campaign for Tobacco-Free Kids. The group aims to stop youth tobacco use. Henigan says, "[Many] kids who use . . . e-cigarette products are using them regularly—twenty days out of a thirty-day month. That's not experimental. That suggests mass addiction."[5]

The third stage is the risky use of a substance. People at this stage crave the

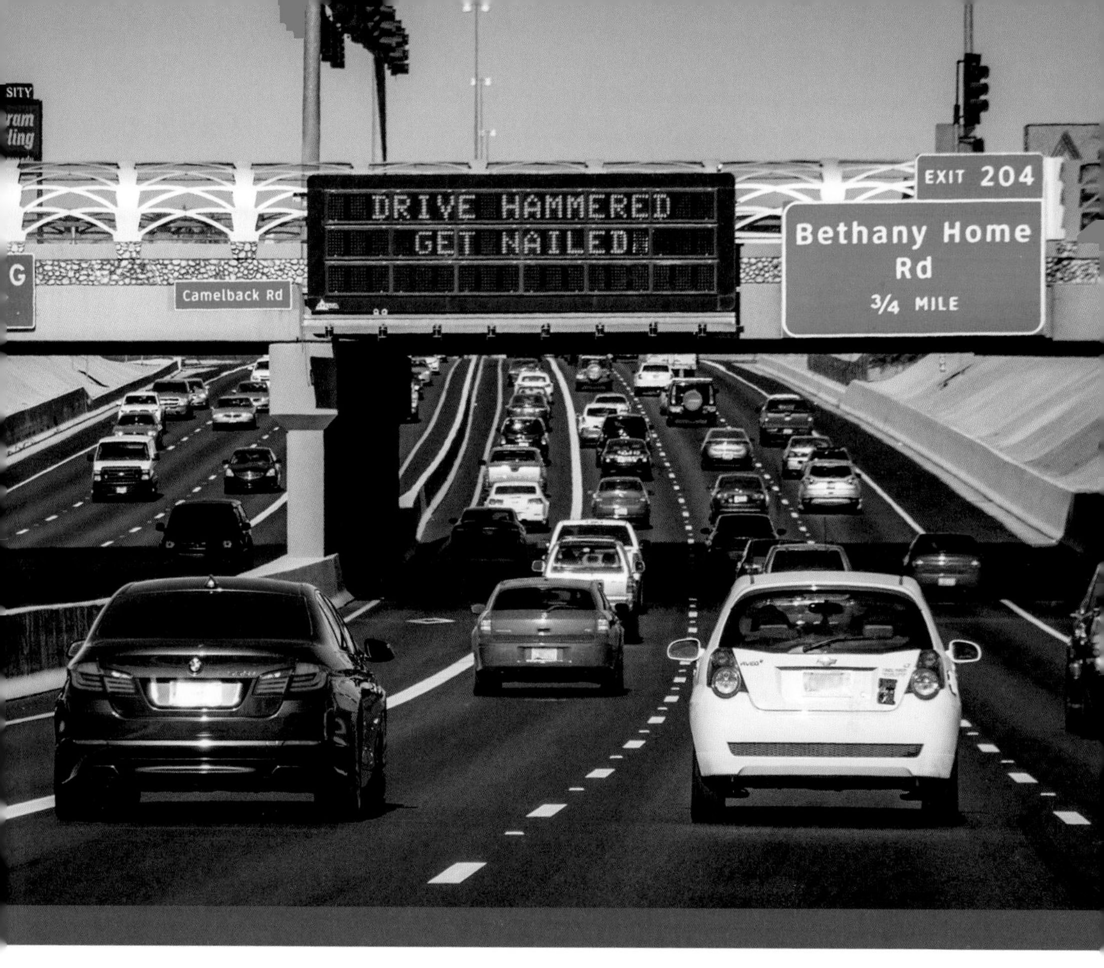

In some cities road signs warn people of the dangers of driving under the influence of alcohol or other substances.

substance more often. They may start to take more risks. They might start to use the substance at school. Or they may steal money to pay for it. People may miss work or break laws. For example, they might drive while drunk.

The fourth stage is dependence. People who depend on drugs use them daily. They may use the drugs many times each day. They develop a tolerance. They may feel sick if they stop using the substance.

People who can no longer control their substance use have an addiction. They use the substance all the time. It is all they can think about. They crave it and seek it out no matter the costs. They may try to stop using the substance. Most people who have addictions cannot stop using substances for long. They may try to stop but relapse, or start using the substances again.

WHY DO PEOPLE USE SUBSTANCES?

Some substances increase the dopamine in a person's brain. Dopamine is a chemical. It sends signals from the brain to the body's

WHAT IS RELAPSE?

Relapse is common among people who have SUDs. The relapse may be triggered by stress. Or people may be around others who are using the substance. They start to think about how they felt the last time they used the substance. They might start to slip back into bad habits. For example, they may avoid other users. They want to remain clean. But they feel an urge to start using again. They begin to give in to these cravings.

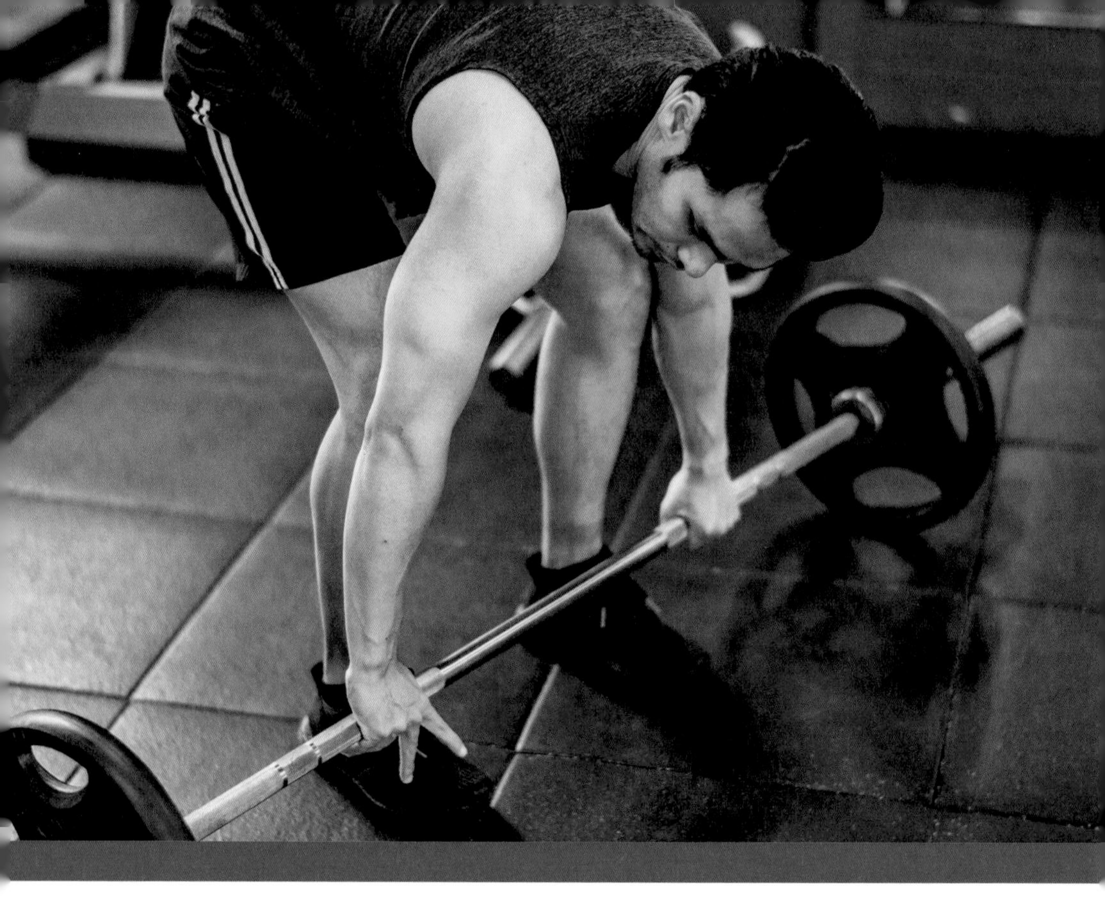

Some people use drugs to improve their academic or athletic performance without considering the risks.

nerve cells. It gives people a sense of pleasure. The more dopamine people have, the better they feel.

The brain releases dopamine as a reward for certain actions. This makes the person want to do these actions more often. The same is true of drugs that release dopamine. People want to continue using the drugs because of this reward. Some drugs ease pain. Others relieve stress.

Peer pressure often plays a role in addiction. Peer pressure is the influence of friends. Friends may pressure others to start using substances. People may feel left out if they do not join in. They may also be curious about what their friends are doing. They want to try it for themselves.

Some people start using substances to improve their performance. For example, students may want to stay awake to study for a test. They may use drugs that make them feel more awake and alert. Steroid abuse is also common. These substances help build muscles. People who compete in sports might abuse steroids.

WHAT ARE THE SYMPTOMS OF AN ADDICTION?

Addiction has many symptoms. The symptoms vary from person to person. They depend on the substance. They also depend on a person's family history and other factors. Not everyone shows all the signs.

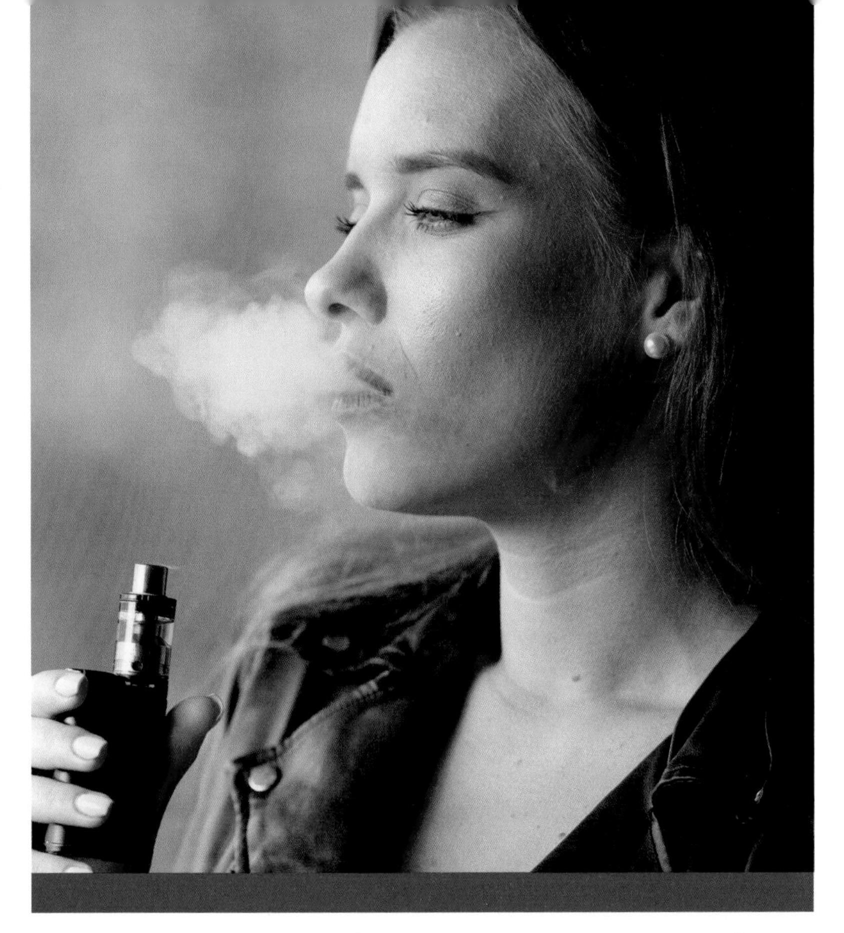

Someone who is addicted to drugs may spend a lot of their free time finding ways to get high.

The most common sign is a constant need for a substance. People spend a lot of time seeking out the substance. They lose interest in anything else. They may avoid going to places where they cannot use the substance. Often they stop doing hobbies such as sports.

People may also try to hide their substance use. Or they may lie about it. This is another sign of addiction. These people do not want others to know about their behavior. They may use the substance alone or in secret.

OTHER EFFECTS OF DRUG USAGE

Drugs can make people hear or see things that are not there. This imaginary experience is called a hallucination. People lose touch with reality. They may develop false ideas or beliefs. They may believe that other people do not like them. Or they may think that others are trying to harm them. Drugs can also make people feel angry.

People who have an SUD often stop taking care of themselves. Substance abuse also changes people's brain chemistry. They may behave in ways that are out of character. They may be moody or angry. They may lash out at loved ones in anger. They are also more likely to take risks. For example, they may drive too fast. Or they may get into fights.

THE CONSEQUENCES OF ADDICTION

Substance abuse can cause health problems. It can affect every organ in the body. The effects depend on the type of substance. They also depend on how much of the substance a person uses. How often a person uses it plays a role too. Doctors use scans and blood tests to see the damage.

Some people use needles to inject drugs into their veins. People may share needles with others. Diseases can be spread in this way. Also, some drugs destroy nerve cells. Or they may cause brain damage. Others damage users' teeth. Smoking can cause breathing difficulties and lung cancer.

Many people who abuse substances have mental health issues. Sometimes these issues exist before the addiction.

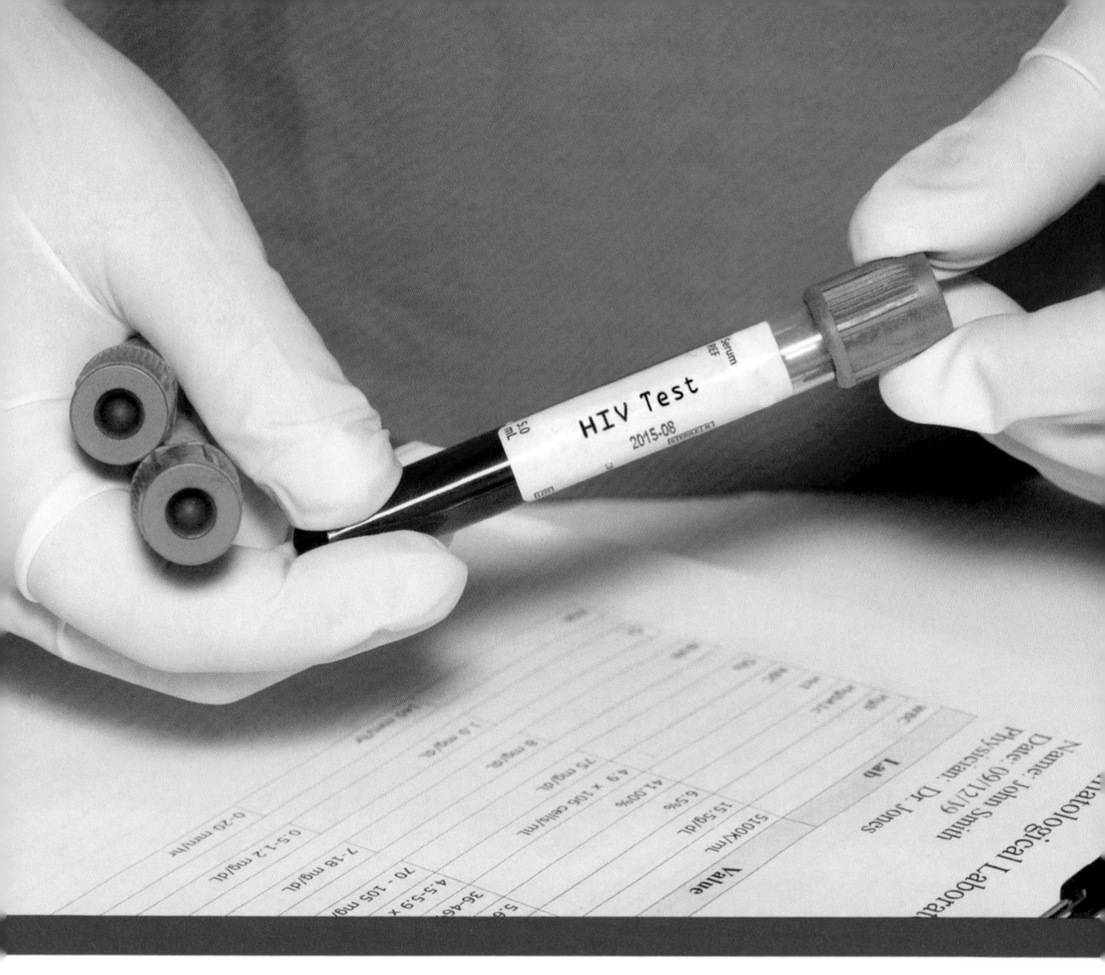

Drug addictions can create health complications. Injecting drugs causes a higher risk of diseases such as HIV or hepatitis.

People use drugs to help them feel better. But drugs can make mental health issues worse. They can make people feel more anxious or depressed.

Money problems often result from addiction. People who have an SUD may have a lot of debt. They borrow money to spend on drugs. They may not have enough money to pay their bills. They may lose their home as a result. They cannot afford to eat healthy meals. Their physical

ROBERT DOWNEY JR.

Robert Downey Jr. is an actor. He starred in the Iron Man movies. He first tried cannabis when he was six years old. His dad gave it to him. Downey was addicted to the drug by the age of eight. He tried all kinds of drugs with his dad. He was arrested many times for risky behavior such as speeding. He finally stopped using drugs in 2003. He went through treatment. The treatment helped him overcome his addiction.

health gets worse. They may be arrested for drug use, theft, or other risky activities.

Substance abuse affects people's relationships as well. People tell lies to hide their substance abuse. They may also miss important family events. They may get angry when others offer to help them find treatment. Many people with an SUD do not know they have a problem. They think they are in control of their substance use. They think they can stop using the substance at any time. They are in **denial**.

CHAPTER THREE

HOW DOES ADDICTION AFFECT SOCIETY?

Substance abuse is one of the top health problems in the United States. It also affects people around the world. Nearly six percent of people around the world use illegal drugs. More than two percent have an SUD.

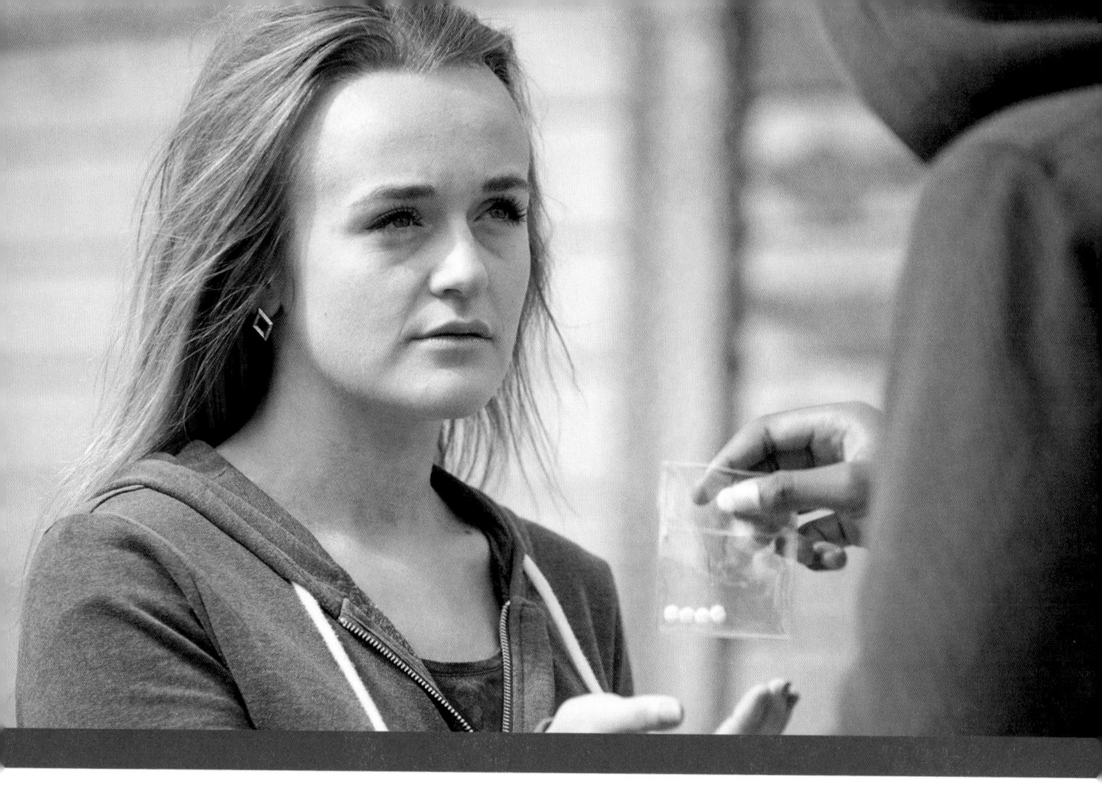

In 2017, 14 percent of young adults between the ages of eighteen and twenty-five reported taking prescription drugs for nonmedical purposes.

SUDs cause many health issues. Governments spend a lot of time and money treating these issues. Health issues caused by SUDs killed nearly 12 million people in 2017. More than half were younger than fifty years old.

ADDICTION IN THE UNITED STATES

More than 20 million Americans over the age of twelve have an SUD. Only about 10 percent of these people get the help they need. There are more drug-related deaths in the United States than in any other wealthy country. More than 67,000 Americans died from drug overdoses in 2018. This was

WHAT IS AN OVERDOSE?

Sometimes people take too much of a drug. Or they mix different drugs together. Their body cannot process the drugs. They become very sick. Some end up in a coma. Others have a heart attack, stroke, or seizure. Many die. This type of death is called an overdose. Most people can be saved if they get medical help in time.

three times higher than in 1999. Overdose is a type of substance abuse. It happens when people take a dangerous amount of a drug.

Nearly half of all US inmates are in prison for drug-related crimes. Every twenty-five seconds, someone is arrested for having drugs. The government spends more than $9 million a day to keep people in jail for these crimes. State governments spend even more. All this money comes from taxpayers.

Substances such as alcohol can affect people's driving. People may

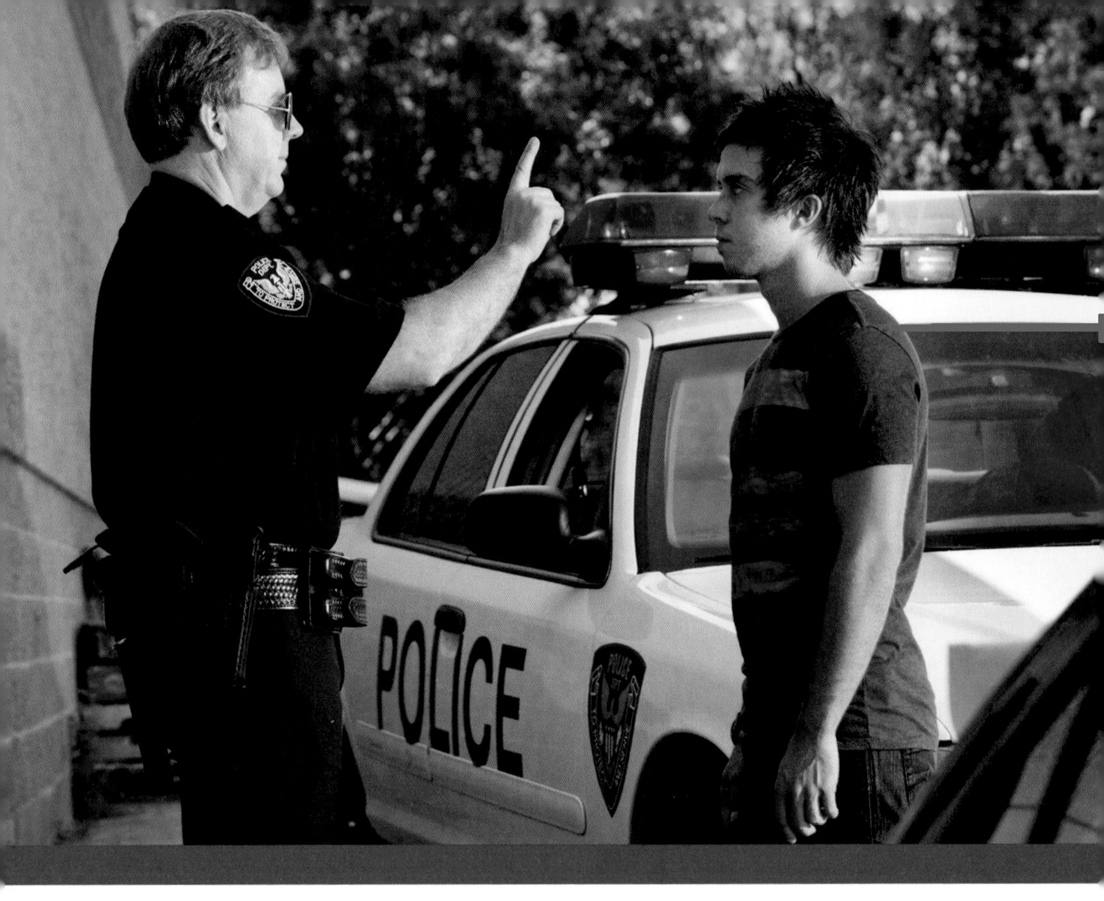

Twenty-nine percent of fatal car accidents in the United States in 2018 were caused by driving under the influence of alcohol.

get in car crashes. They may end up killing themselves or others. About thirty Americans die in alcohol-related car crashes each day. That is about one person every forty-eight minutes.

There are many costs related to substance abuse. These costs involve crime, health care, and job loss. Substance abuse can also lead to homelessness and accidents. The United States spends $700 billion each year in these areas.

HOW DOES ADDICTION AFFECT CHILDREN?

About one in eight US children lives with at least one parent who has an SUD. Addiction can affect the parents' ability to care for their children. The parents may put their need for the substance first. They may spend most of their money on drugs. There may not be much money left over to take care of their children's needs. Parents who have an SUD may **neglect** their children. They can only think about how to get more of a substance. As a result, their children often do not get proper health and dental care. Their kids

SUBSTANCE ABUSE AND HOMELESSNESS

More than 560,000 Americans were homeless in 2019. Many homeless people have addictions. They face harsh living conditions on the streets. Many also have mental health issues. Some were homeless before they developed an SUD. They began using substances to cope. Others are homeless because of their substance abuse.

may not have enough food or proper clothing. The parents and their children may become homeless.

David Sheff is an author. He writes about addiction. His son has an SUD. He says, “If a parent had a heart problem or cancer . . . it’d be talked about in school with teachers.”[6] He points out that people often offer help with childcare in these cases. Many also bring food to the person’s family. But this is usually not the case when someone has a parent with an SUD. Sheff says, “The child is shamed. There’s no sense of community support.”[7]

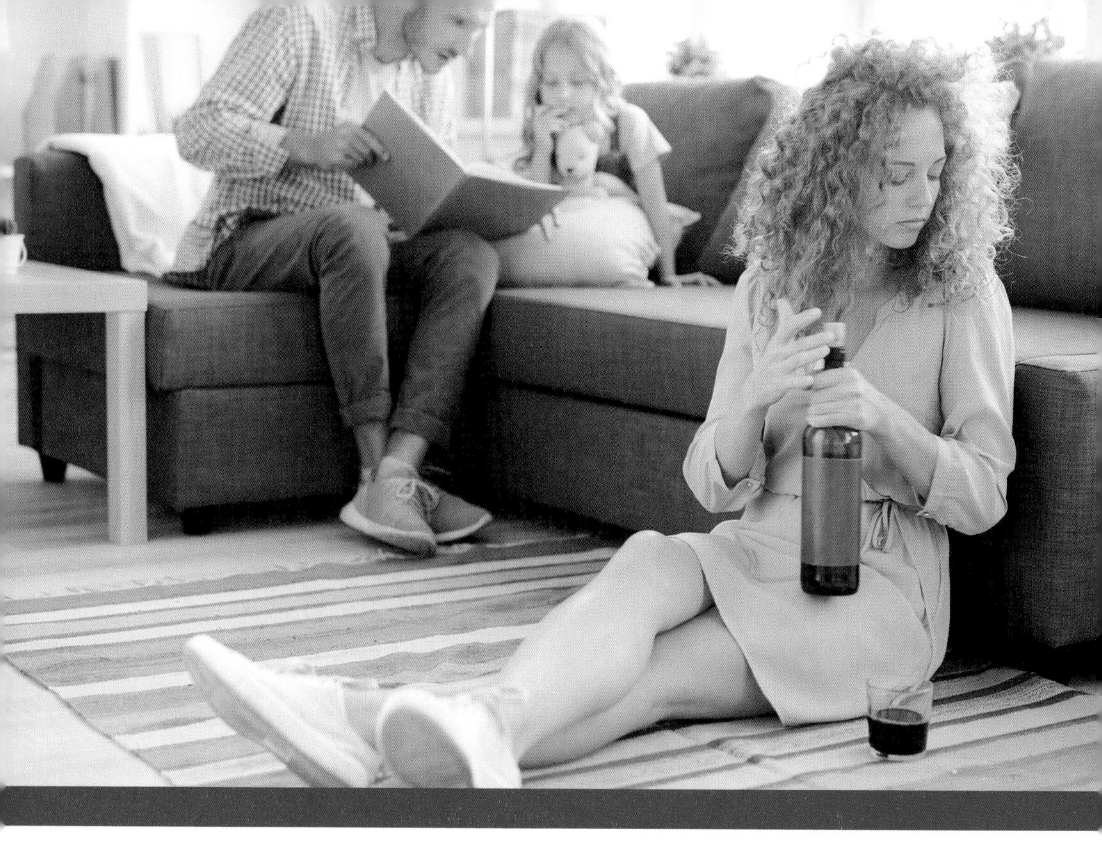

A parent who has an SUD might be less engaged in their child's school and other activities.

Shame often feeds into addiction. People who feel ashamed have low self-esteem. They may think they are worthless. The shame may come from their upbringing. A parent may have neglected or abused them. As a result, they may feel unloved.

They might start using substances to make themselves feel better. Then they might develop an addiction.

HOW DOES ADDICTION AFFECT BUSINESSES?

Addiction can affect people's ability to do their jobs. They often miss work or come in late. They also may not get along well with others. Their cravings may make them irritable. Their coworkers have to work harder to make up for their lack of effort.

People who do not have enough money to buy drugs may become desperate. Some steal money from their workplace.

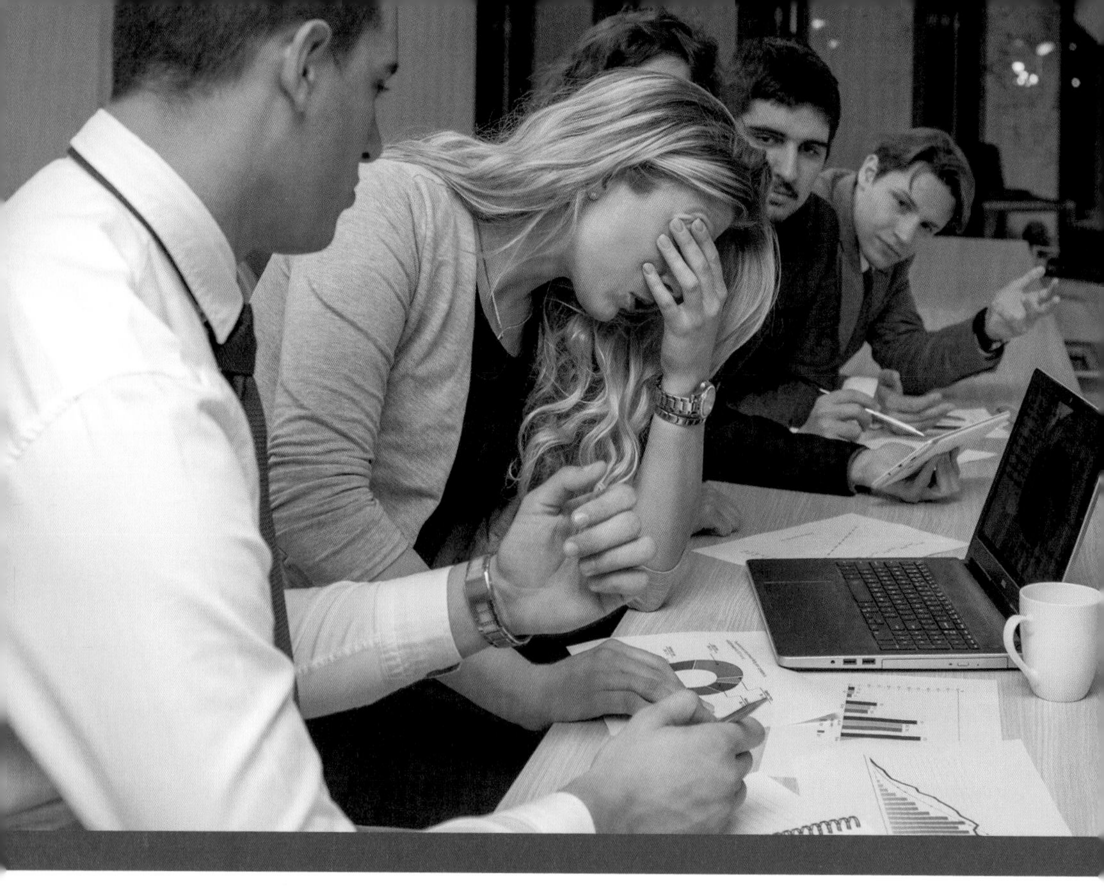

Employees who struggle with addiction are often less productive. This can cause issues with coworkers.

Others steal work supplies or equipment. They sell these items to get drug money. People with SUDs may also find it hard to focus on work tasks. They think only about the next time they will be able to use the substance. They get less work done than their coworkers. They make mistakes in their work. Companies lose money due to substance abuse issues such as theft and lost productivity.

Some people with an SUD have dangerous jobs. For example, they may be construction workers. They may operate heavy machinery. Mistakes on the job can put people at risk. People can cause accidents. This can lead to injuries or deaths. Many companies pay for part of their employees' health insurance. These costs are higher for employees who have an SUD. This is because these people often require more health care.

Kirt Walker works for Nationwide. Nationwide is an insurance company. Walker thinks companies should pay for proper addiction treatment. This can help companies save money in the long term. Some companies fire workers who have addictions. Then they hire new workers. But it is cheaper to take care of current employees than to train new ones. Walker says, "Addiction is a workforce issue. If business leaders can . . . get people the help they need while keeping

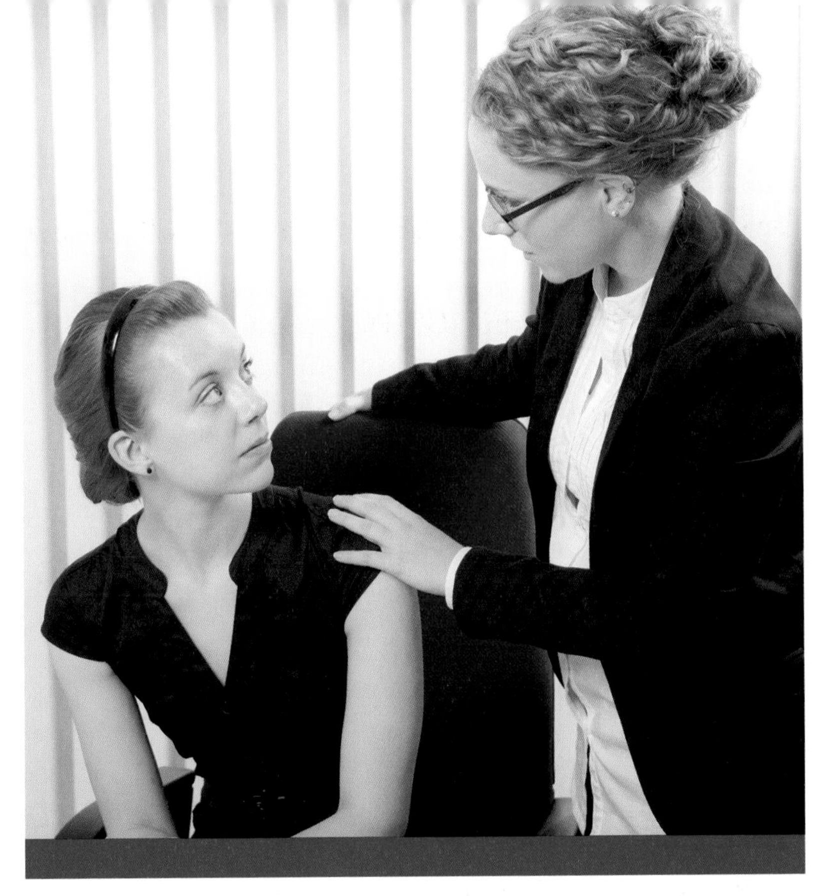

Studies have shown that when companies provide resources to help their employees with addiction, the employees' productivity increases.

them employed, it could make a huge difference."[8] He adds that employees may be more loyal to companies that offer this help. They will be better workers after they have gone through treatment.

CHAPTER FOUR

HOW IS ADDICTION TREATED?

There is no cure for addiction. But it can be treated. However, people may not seek treatment right away. Many people feel ashamed of their SUD. They may not know where to go for help. Or they may feel hopeless. They may not think it is possible to overcome their addiction.

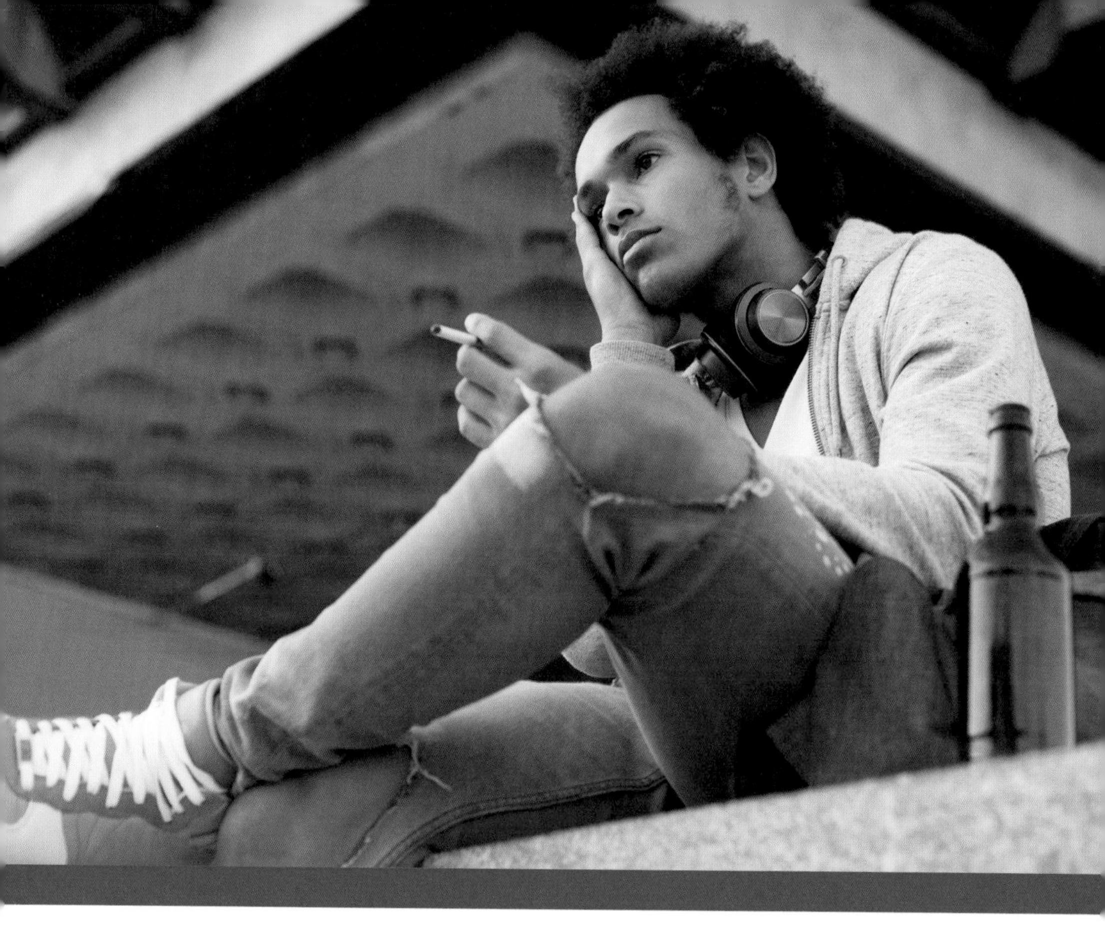

Only about 20 percent of people who have an SUD receive treatment.

People who have their addiction under control are said to be in recovery. The first step to recovery is admitting there is a problem. Then people may be motivated to seek treatment. Rehabilitation programs, or rehab, can help. Mental health professionals run these programs. They are trained to help people overcome addiction.

THERAPY

Therapy is part of most treatment plans. Some mental health professionals are trained to provide therapy. They are called therapists. People meet with therapists to talk about their addiction. They may meet daily. Or they may meet many times each week. People talk about what is going on in their life. They discuss their feelings and relationships. They talk about people or situations that cause stress.

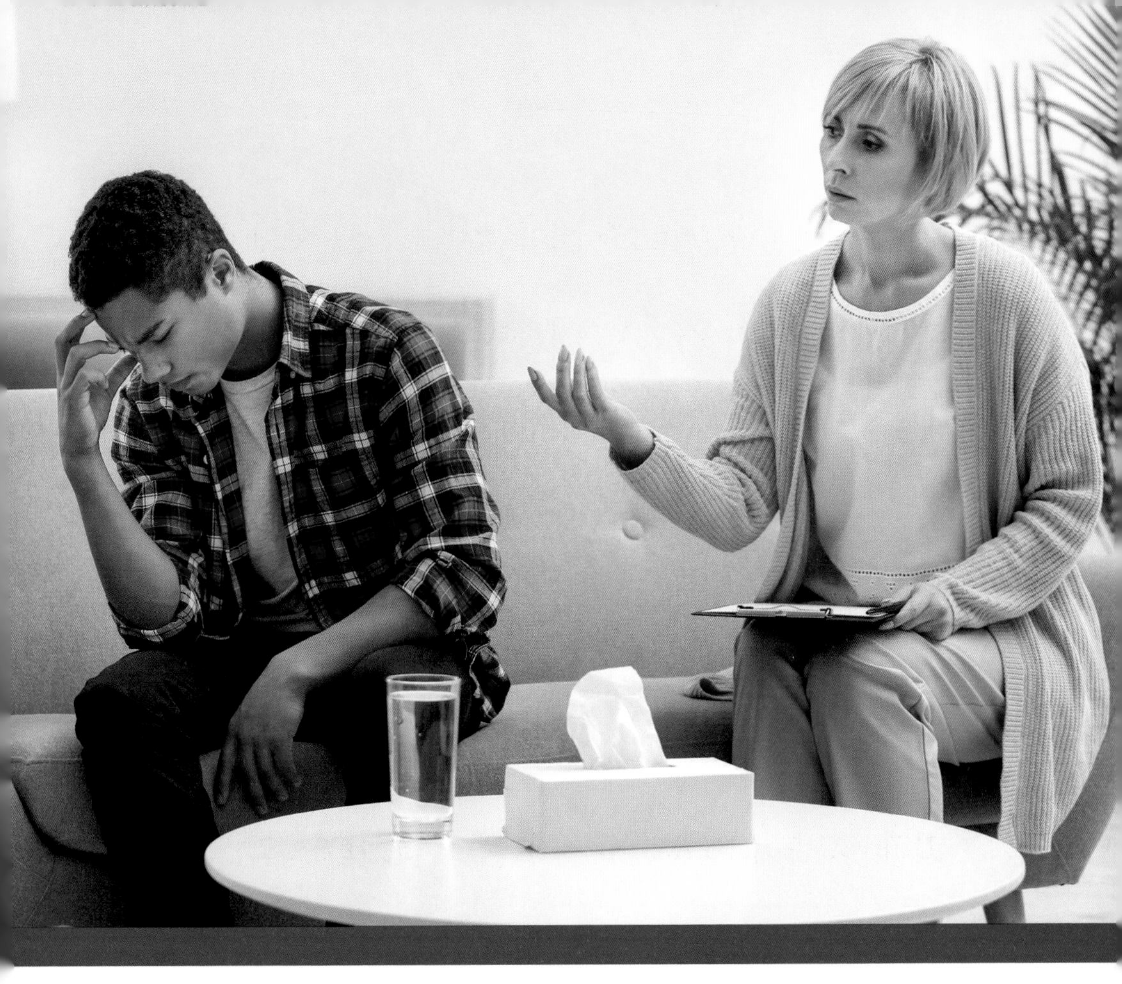

Behavioral therapy helps people create coping strategies. They learn how to recognize environments or events that could trigger cravings for the drug.

Behavioral therapy is often helpful for people who have an addiction. It is based on the idea that all behaviors are learned. This means that a behavior can change.

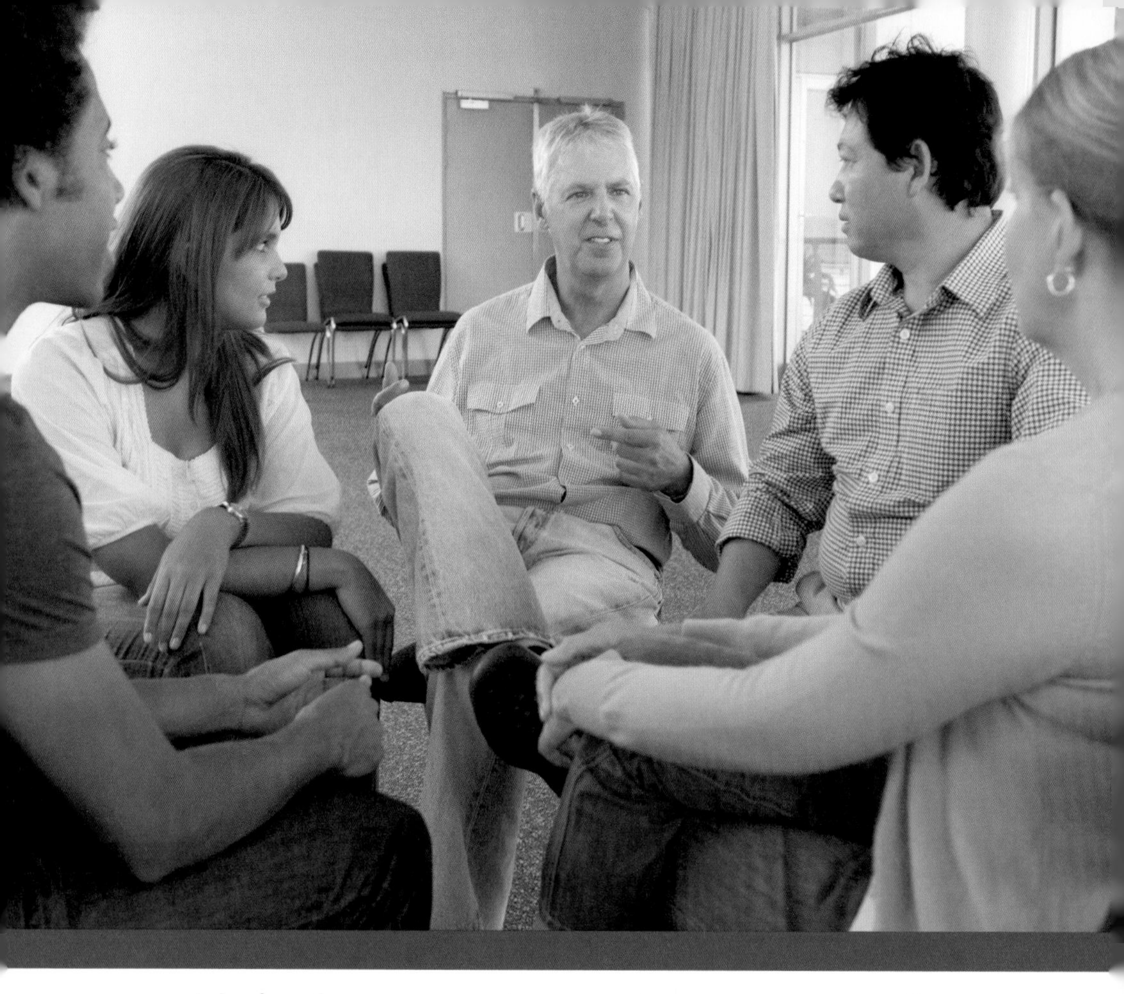

A trained person leads group therapy sessions. The leader encourages and guides people to be open about their struggles so they do not feel isolated during their recovery.

Therapists help people see how their thoughts affect their actions. They teach how to spot unhealthy behaviors. People learn healthy ways to deal with stress.

They work to change their thoughts and actions. They learn how to ask for help.

Some people meet with therapists individually. They may also go to group therapy. In group therapy, a therapist meets with a group of people. The people struggle with similar issues. Group therapy helps people realize they are not alone. They see that others share their experiences.

INPATIENT PROGRAMS

Rehab is a treatment process. It helps restore people's health. There are many types of programs. No single program is right for everyone. It is important for people

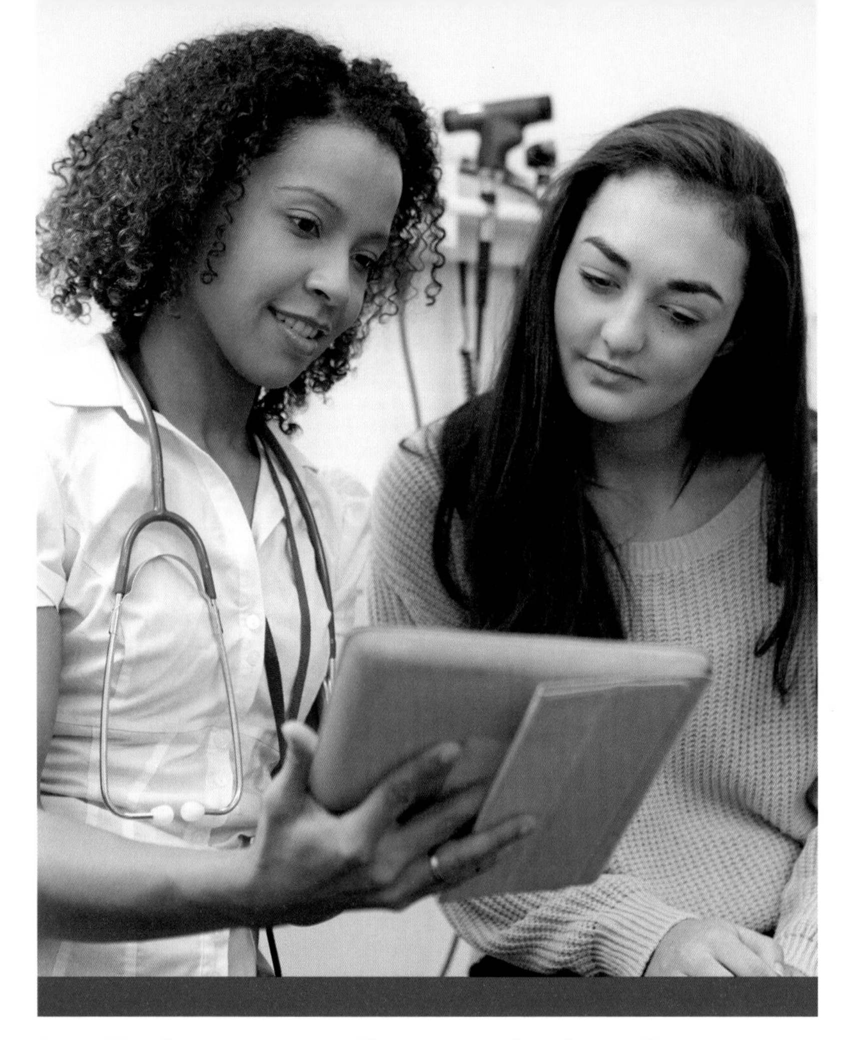

Inpatient programs allow people struggling with addiction to stay in a safe environment with constant medical and emotional support from professionals.

to find which works best for them. The program should meet their needs. It may include more than one type of treatment.

Inpatient programs can help people who have SUDs. These programs are offered at treatment centers. People live in a treatment center for a period of time. Most stay at the center for thirty, sixty, or ninety days. But some stay as long as six months. They get medical care. They attend daily therapy sessions too.

Inpatient programs can help people who have relapsed. They also work well for people who come from high-risk environments. For example, some people might live with a loved one who also has an SUD. Or they may have other challenges in their home environment. They might have money troubles or easy access to drugs.

Some people have bad withdrawal symptoms. Withdrawal happens when people stop using a substance. Their body depends on the substance. They get sick without it. Doctors in inpatient

RELAPSE

Relapse is a common setback. People may be substance-free for months or years. Then something stressful could happen. For example, a loved one may die. People may begin using substances again to cope. About 40 to 60 percent of people relapse within the first year of treatment.

NDC 12496-1208-3
30 pouches each containing
1 sublingual film
8 mg/2 mg
Suboxone®
(buprenorphine and naloxone) sublingual film
8 mg/2 mg
Rx only
Children who accidentally take SUBOXONE will need emergency medical care. Keep SUBOXONE out of the reach of children.
Do not cut, chew or swallow sublingual film.
suboxone.com

Suboxone can be prescribed to help relieve symptoms of withdrawal from opioids.

programs can treat people when they go through withdrawal.

OUTPATIENT PROGRAMS

Outpatient programs are another type of treatment. They offer the same services as inpatient programs. But people do not live at the treatment center. They are free to leave each day. They can go to school or work. They come back to the center at a time that works for them. Some people go to the center every day. Others go a few times a week.

Outpatient programs vary in length. Some last three months. Others last more than one year. People usually spend ten to twelve hours per week at the treatment center.

DETOXIFICATION

Most treatment plans start with detoxification, or detox. Detox involves

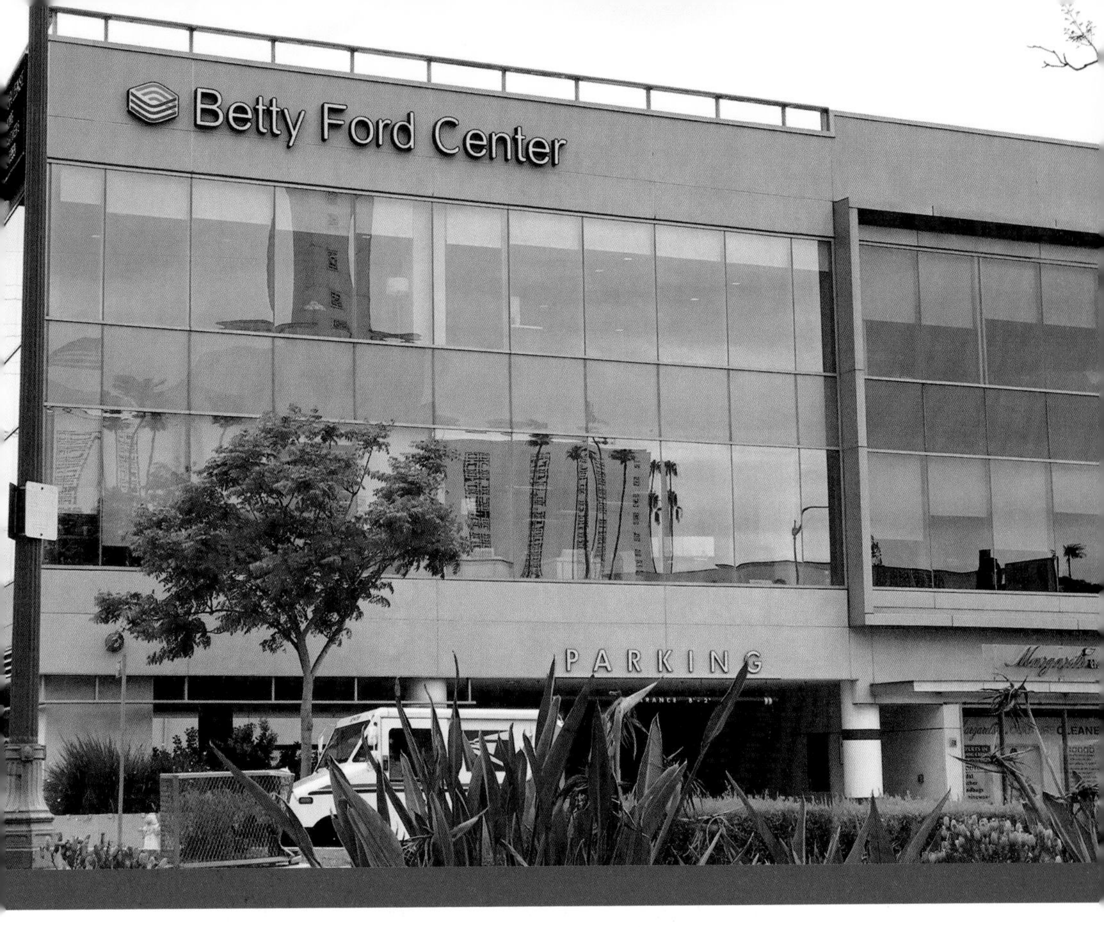

The detox process can be very dangerous. Treatment centers, such as this one, have programs to help people detox safely.

clearing out all addictive substances from a person's body. It often takes a few days to a week. This process should be done under the care of health workers. People should never try to detox by themselves.

Detox is often painful. People may have bad withdrawal symptoms. They may get headaches. They shake and sweat a lot. They may feel anxious or depressed. Memory and sleep problems are common too. Some people develop severe health

WHAT IS AN INTERVENTION?

Some families and friends plan an intervention. This is a meeting with someone who has an SUD. The person may be in denial. He may not think he needs help. Loved ones encourage the person to seek help. They talk with the person about the addiction. They show that they care about the person's well-being. They also let the person know that they will help with the recovery process. Professionals can help people plan interventions.

problems when they detox. They may have seizures. Doctors provide medications to help reduce withdrawal symptoms.

People who try to detox by themselves could die. They need proper treatment during this period. The risk of relapse is also higher when people do not have help. People may start using the substance again to feel better.

SUPPORT GROUPS

Many people join support groups to help manage their addiction. People who have an alcohol addiction may go to an Alcoholics Anonymous (AA) group.

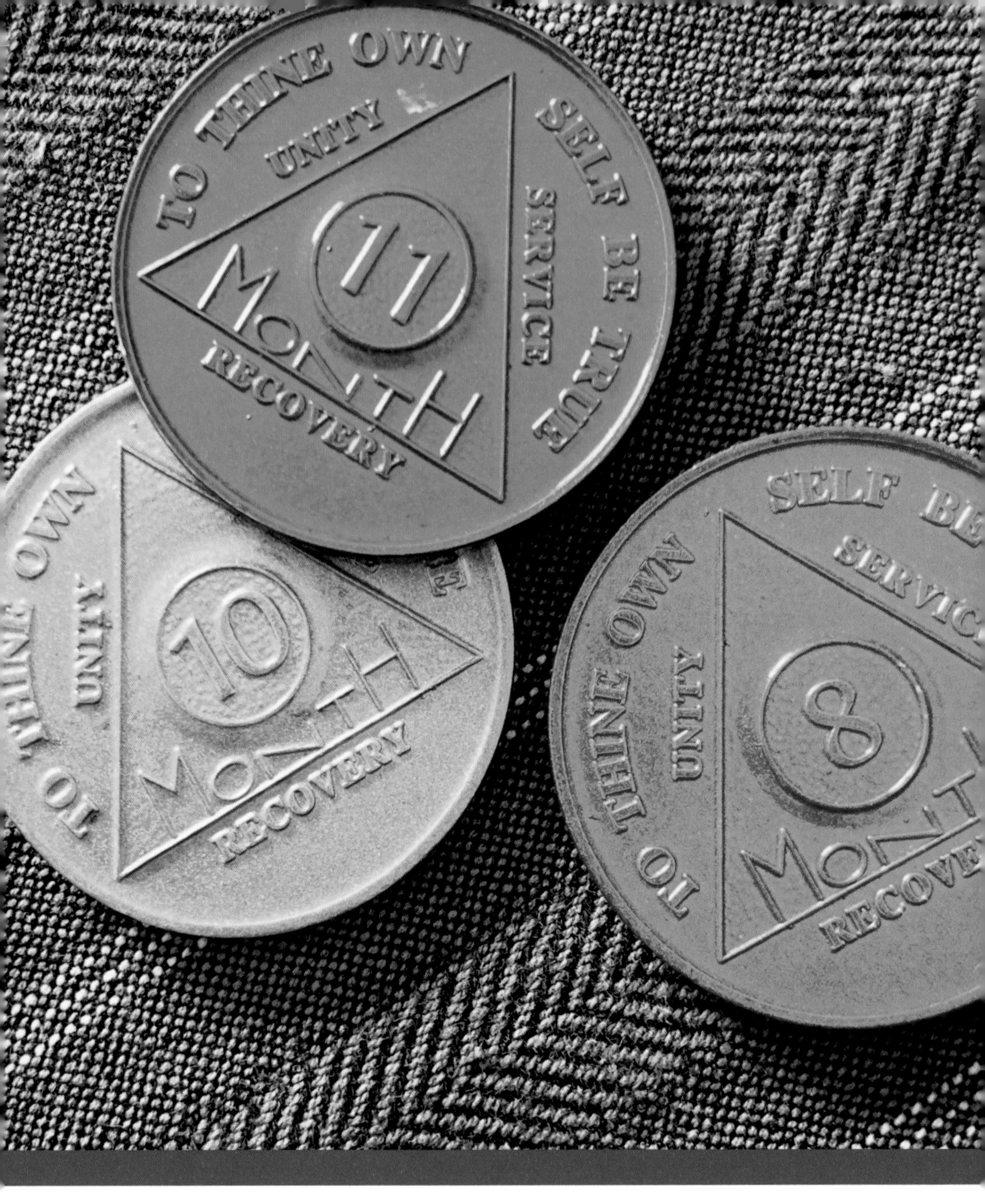

Members of Alcoholics Anonymous (AA) are given a sobriety token for each month they remain substance free.

Those who have a drug addiction may go to a Narcotics Anonymous (NA) group. There are many AA and NA groups throughout the country. These groups meet many times each week. People can go to as many meetings as they want. The groups provide a safe and welcoming environment. People talk about their experiences and their recovery. Nothing people say is shared outside the meeting.

Family or friends of people who have SUDs often need support too. Their lives are affected by their loved ones' addictions. There are support groups available to them.

Al-Anon groups help people whose loved ones are addicted to alcohol. Nar-Anon groups help people whose loved ones are addicted to drugs.

HOPE FOR THE FUTURE

Addiction often lasts many years. It can cause many health problems. But treatment can prevent further health damage. It can help people recover.

Ryan Hess had an SUD for fifteen years. He thought there was no hope for recovery. Then one day he asked for help. He went through treatment. He did not think he could repair his relationships. He also did not think he could get his job back or buy a home. But he was able to do all these things. He says, “It’s hard work . . . but today life is amazing.”[9]

DEMI LOVATO

Demi Lovato is a singer and actress. She has struggled with substance abuse. She began using drugs in 2009. She was seventeen years old. She went into an inpatient program the next year. But she relapsed in 2012. She relapsed again in 2018. Each time, she went through treatment. Lovato says, “If you’ve relapsed . . . just know it’s possible to take that step towards recovery. If you’re alive today, you can make it back. You’re worth it.”

Quoted in Sabrina Barr, “Demi Lovato Shares Powerful Message About Relapse on Instagram,” Independent, *March 16, 2019. www.independent.co.uk.*

GLOSSARY

cannabis

a drug, often called marijuana, that is made from the cannabis plant

coma

a state of being unconscious or unable to wake that can last a long time and is caused by brain damage

denial

when people refuse to believe or accept that something is true

neglect

to not give enough care or attention to something or to ignore it

prescription

orders from a doctor to give a person certain medications

seizure

a condition that happens when there is a lot of electrical activity in the brain, which often makes people shake uncontrollably

stressed

the feeling created by the body's response to demands

tolerance

the ability to handle more of a substance without it having any effects

SOURCE NOTES

INTRODUCTION: THE PATH TO ADDICTION

1. "True Story: Alex," *Phoenix House*, August 28, 2014. www.phoenixhouse.org.

CHAPTER ONE: WHAT IS ADDICTION?

2. Quoted in Taylor Bennett, "What Does Addiction Feel Like?" *ThriveWorks*, August 10, 2018. www.thriveworks.com.

3. Quoted in Brittany Risher, "The Truth About Whether Vaping Is Safer than Smoking Cigarettes," *Prevention*, November 2, 2018. www.prevention.com.

CHAPTER TWO: HOW DOES ADDICTION AFFECT PEOPLE?

4. Quoted in Beth Leipholtz, "The Four Stages of Addiction," *Orlando Recovery Center*, n.d. www.orlandorecoverycenter.com.

5. Quoted in Dennis Thompson, "What Works to Help Teens Quit Vaping?" *WebMD*, January 31, 2019. www.webmd.com.

CHAPTER THREE: HOW DOES ADDICTION AFFECT SOCIETY?

6. Quoted in Alana Levinson, "Surviving the Secret Childhood Trauma of a Parent's Drug Addiction," *Pacific Standard*, June 14, 2017. www.psmag.com.

7. Quoted in Levinson, "Surviving the Secret Childhood Trauma."

8. Kirt Walker, "Addiction Is a Workforce Issue. Here's How Business Leaders Can Address It," *Fortune*, November 13, 2019. www.fortune.com.

CHAPTER FOUR: HOW IS ADDICTION TREATED?

9. Quoted in Alexandra Rockey Fleming, "After Hitting 'Rock Bottom,' Some Addicts and Alcoholics Find a Road to Recovery," *Washington Post*, February 23, 2019. www.washingtonpost.com.

WEBSITES

Alcoholics Anonymous (AA)

www.aa.org

Learn more about AA and how it helps people who have substance use disorders.

Child Mind Institute

https://childmind.org

This site offers resources about risk factors and many other topics related to mental health. It can help people learn more about SUDs.

MentalHealth.gov

www.mentalhealth.gov

This website provides information about mental health and SUDs.

The Substance Abuse and Mental Health Services Administration (SAMHSA)

www.samhsa.gov

The SAMHSA shares information and resources for people with SUDs. People can learn more about SUDs and related mental health issues. The SAMHSA also provides a helpline number.

INDEX

IMAGE CREDITS

Cover: © TheVisualsYouNeed/Shutterstock Images
5: © alacatr/iStockphoto
7: © Dmytro Tyshchenko/Shutterstock Images
8: © Africa Studio/Shutterstock Images
11: © SpeedKingz/Shutterstock Images
13: © PabloBenitezLope/iStockphoto
16: © AndreyPopov/iStockphoto
21: © Red Line Editorial
25: © iordani/Shutterstock Images
26: © fotoNino/Shutterstock Images
29: © melissamn/Shutterstock Images
32: © Auttapol Sangsub/Shutterstock Images
35: © sestovic/iStockphoto
39: © Sherry Yates Young/Shutterstock Images
43: © SpeedKingz/Shutterstock Images
46: © DarrenMower/iStockphoto
50: © shironosov/iStockphoto
52: © zoff-photo/iStockphoto
55: © Sebastian Gauert/Shutterstock Images
57: © Prostock-studio/Shutterstock Images
59: © New Africa/Shutterstock Images
60: © Monkey Business Images/Shutterstock Images
62: © Monkey Business Images/Shutterstock Images
65: © PureRadiancePhoto/Shutterstock Images
67: © Alex Millauer/Shutterstock Images
70: © Lorenza Ochoa/Shutterstock Images

ABOUT THE AUTHOR

Heather C. Hudak has written hundreds of books for children. She writes about all kinds of topics, from natural disasters to world events. When she's not writing, Heather enjoys traveling all over the world. She has visited more than fifty countries. She also loves camping in the mountains near her home with her husband and their many rescue cats and dogs.